Farming Broke Me, But I Keep Fighting

Thriving not just surviving

Leanne Barriball

Farming Broke Me, But I keep Fighting

All views expressed in this publication are the authors own, through her own personal experiences. They are not to be reprinted or shared without prior consent of the author.

Where quoting about Neuroscience, Neuro-coaching this information has been obtained through Dr Shannon Irvine, who the author trained under to get a SINC Neuro-coaching Qualification. Any further information can be found on her website.

Copyright © 2024 Leanne Barriball
All Rights Reserved
ISBN: 9798333757838
Imprint: Independently published

Dedication:

I dedicate this book to my family, who have seen me go and grow through this entire journey and have supported me every single step of the way. I will be forever grateful I ended up in this family, because I am right where I am supposed to be.

FOREWORD

This short book is Leanne's honest and inspiring account of how she found a better way to think and live, guided by God and Neuroscience. She gives such a profound account of how she came to her new approach to life that I am sure many people will find themselves thinking that they can associate with some of the mental and physical states she describes. I see Leanne apply her new ways of thinking in her daily life, in motherhood, farming and business, and I know that she inspires others in her life. I am sure that after reading her book you too will want to rewire your brain to embrace the changes you want to see in your own lives.

PROLOGUE

How to write a book? The truth is I have no real idea, all I know is, I want to share what I have learnt so far, and a book seems the simplest way to do that. I shall make a start and we shall see where we end up.

Once upon a time, only kidding it's not going to be one of those kinds of books, I'm not quite at my happy ever after, but I am living happier than I was before. Before what? I hear you say, before I became a mum, before I fully understood my own mind and body. I am no longer running a farming business with a body that didn't want to work anymore. My mind and body are now healing. This book is my explanation of how I found a way to thrive in farming and in life.

CHAPTER ONE

I have a message to share which I believe can help people, and a short blog post, video, or conversation just won't get my whole point across. So, as I write I am going to imagine we are sitting in my sitting-room and we are chatting. Now if you are a friend of mine who has sat in my sitting room, some of the situations I share with you will be familiar with, but a lot you won't, because I have been learning all these things about myself quietly in the background, knowing and trusting that one day my story will make a difference in the lives of others. I know this because the chances are if you are reading this, something is going to resonate with you, and I hope and pray that you will find a different or even new perspective. A perspective that opens your eyes to the possibilities of what could happen when you start to seek a healthier, happier life for you and your family.

A bit of background, I was the eldest to be born in the 5th generation of our farming family. Our farm is on the Devon and Cornwall border on the Devon side at Lifton, we have cows, sheep, goats, chickens, pigs, cats, dogs, guinea pigs and anything else which happens to turn up since Covid year! Before it was just cows and sheep. We are also very blessed to have a mile of the river Tamar all to ourselves. One minute we can be in Devon, the next in Cornwall.

It was my dad's family farm, and my mum was bought up in a family where her dad was a farm worker. She was therefore very aware of the work ethic of farmers, mainly being to work away for 365 days of the year, in all weathers at all times of the day. Hoping that one day you get lucky and make a fortune farming, and it all becomes easier. "Make a fortune in farming", that's laughable for sure! I've since learnt that this theory hasn't worked for a long time, and it's the decisions and actions I make daily towards our farming business that determines whether the business will work or not, whether we will still even have a farm in 20 years time if things carry on as they have.

Our farm business should be here to help to pay for our living, keep the roof over our heads, and food on the table. Not destroy my health, which is what happened to me. It used to be a farm could support 3 or 4 families, in the last 30 years that's changed massively as has the state of the UK.

I have a younger brother, and we were brought up with the help of both sets of grandparents, this is something of a rarity now. The difference being my grandparents were retired, but my parents now are still working so it's not been so easy to call on them for help bringing up our daughter. As of writing this I only have one granny left, and she has been through the mill herself with her mental and physical health, again a girl coming from a farming family. More importantly she was the 5th girl in the farming family before the much sort after boys were born. She has struggled her entire life with so many things, because she never got the help she needed back when she needed it. That's because mental health was still so much of a taboo subject, you just got shipped off to a mental asylum and dosed up with suppressant drugs no questions asked. We have had to walk dear granny through 2 more hospital stays in my lifetime, and after 50 years she can finally say she has a better quality of life because she is able to have better relationships with us all.

Up until about the age of 19 I wanted to be anywhere else but on our farm, constantly wanting to run away, working all the hours I could in pubs, cafes, and shops to avoid the inevitable fact that I was going to end up farming. Things didn't really change until I married my husband Andrew and we went to New Zealand in 2012 for our honeymoon. We had been away for a month, and I for the first time ever, longed to see the view at home that I had seen for 20 years and took no notice of at all, and had zero appreciation of. Andrew my husband brought a brand-new perspective, because he had never had his own farm, but had always known he was going to be a farmer, watching his dad work on farms as a child. He made me realise I had been born blessed as a farmer's daughter, and if I really thought about it, I didn't want to live anywhere else even if I thought I did sometimes.

It would have been fine if I had been encouraged to stay home farming, instead of being told often "don't come home farming, there is no money in it". "Go and do something else". I was all geared up to go and study to be a paramedic, I had done my heavy goods licence to drive the ambulance, loads of hours volunteering in hospitals, but it wasn't meant to be. In the summer of 2007 grandad passed away incredibly suddenly.

One minute he was in the kitchen talking, and the next minute I had a phone call to say that he had been found dead down by our river. Death is never a good thing, but out of all the people who have passed on from this life, his death was the most traumatic, because I didn't get to say good-bye. He had been working alongside my dad on the farm, so things really did change for all of us.

Sudden early death in farming families happens more often than you would think, considering we should be some of the healthiest people on the planet. Good food, fresh air, lots of exercise. Yet we are seeing it more and more in the industry, sometimes due to accidents, other times just due to chronic stress causing heart attacks and strokes. Then sadly there are those who take their own lives because they cannot see a way out of the difficulties they might find themselves in. For poor old grandad it was the stress that killed him, heart attack or stroke they weren't sure. But at 67 and only 2 years into retirement, it was too soon. I never wanted that to happen again, and I think it's why I have been so hell bent on working out what is stressful in our farming business, and making sure we make changes if we can, to alleviate some of those problems.

You could say farming was and is my destiny! Who am I to run in the opposite direction of the greater plan for my life? Farming always was part of it, I didn't choose to be put in this family but I believe God did.

He put me right here, right now. And that is why I am sharing my story, because my passion is to see people healthier and happier in this life. Not be reliant on medication or doctors to be healthy, but rather discover what it is their body and mind does, and how it can become stronger and healthier using the power of our minds. You too can enjoy every second with your children, have amazing relationships, and a full and active life.

This is the piece of my life I choose to do, helping other women in farming, to start to make positive changes in their farming families. I want to share my knowledge and experiences to show you that there is a purpose for your life especially in farming. Farming is the backbone of the country. I want farming women to succeed, and it is easier to learn from someone else's mistakes and glean from their experience rather than trying to do things alone. If things do not work out as planned, it can force you to give up prematurely. Giving up is just something I don't ever want to do, even though I have said it multiple times, I never give in. Giving up is not an option for farmers, we are needed now, we will be needed in the future. Everyone needs food, and we need it to be better quality over quantity.

CHAPTER TWO

When I look back, I can see things in my life were all building to this point. You could say I've been prepared to reveal a new message, that might just change some lives. Do you know what, I was born in a very blessed situation when it comes to our beautiful farm, labelled as the lands of God, I have always had what I needed. We are richly blessed in so many ways, but especially with our family and the relationships we are cultivating with each other many of which are fairly new. Like the one I now have with my dad. When we are working business ideas out together, I have come to realise our new relationship is far more important than how much money is or isn't in the bank. Relationships whether blood or chosen are what make us truly rich, these are the people we go through life with that make everything we choose to do important. I wanted to make my mum and dad's life easier, so it wasn't so stressful for them. Which I have recently realised I have succeeded in doing so. In turn I have made things easier for myself as well.

I just like you, didn't get to where I am now without a whole lot of physical hardship and pain. Suffering is something everyone goes through in some way, it's what you do with that suffering that counts. What we focus on is what we create. I had physical pain and lots of it, but the reality is it was my mental and emotional pain causing the biggest problems.

This was manifested in my body in 2013 as I was not able to walk unaided. I had learnt to suppress my emotions, knowing only real anger came from the constant fears that I was telling myself all the time. "I wasn't good enough, I was lazy, useless, I didn't fit in, I was too fat". My soul had many open wounds that needed healing. I think I just hoped I could forget things and put them to the back of my mind, how wrong I was. I will share something with you now, it's a whole lot more painful dealing with those thoughts than what it would have been had I have been able to process it properly as a child, or teen and even an adult.

We now know a lot more about the human brain, our thoughts and emotions, than we did when I was growing up, and it's not now for me to keep condemning myself for things that have happened and the way I have treated myself. I didn't know how to set emotional boundaries, I didn't know how to control my temper, I didn't even know that the majority of my thought life was taking up so much of my energy. It was literally preventing me from doing useful normal daily things.

Now I do know that it is possible to change anything and everything in my life I don't particularly like, and things really started to change when I discovered Jesus. I can honestly say that although the road to recovery has been hard and taken longer than I wanted it too, the recovery I will have at the end of this will far surpass any recovery I could have tried to do by myself. I have needed steps to know what to do to get better and these came when I learnt how to be a Neuro coach.

A divine appointment in the right place meant that I was able to literally hold every thought captive like the bible tells us to do. When I used to read that scripture, I had no idea how to do it, yet from my health's perspective it's what I needed to do. We create our lives with our thoughts, if our thoughts are chaotic, harmful, dark, and oppressive, this will show up in our lives. If our thoughts are true, noble, right, pure, lovely, admirable, excellent or praiseworthy, we really can start to experience the goodness of God in the land of the living. Our minds need to be trained to do this though, because we live in a negatively bias world, a world governed by fear which seeks to steal, kill and destroy us, through anxiety and stress.

Up until recently I didn't know how to hold every thought captive, and now I do and it's a joy to be able to offer the same help to others, to get them on the journey to health using a brain-based approach, so inside out rather than outside in which is what many other programs and solutions offer.

As you read this, I want you to realise that everything I write is from experience, I have not gone and learnt about these things from books and then decided to write about them. The truth is there are a whole heap of things that I still want to happen within my life which haven't yet happened. Yet being the key word here, because I believe they will. For example, I have not lost the weight that I know I carry and is not good for my mobility, or my morale. I haven't made my first million yet writing books and coaching clients with their health. What I have done though is learnt to be an amazing mum to my daughter Hayley even if I have yet to find her instruction book. Parenting is like a bloody minefield; you get over one problem and walk right into another. And we have got our farming business to a place of stability for the future so much so I can see the future of us being here, and all the amazing things we are going to see happen and are already happening. From new life coming into the soil and surrounding environment, less work with the animals as their health improves, creating a top quality grass fed product and managing the farm as a business which serves us, rather than us serving it. I am an entrepreneur at heart and we have all sorts of different business ideas popping up, I am one of the few who is actually using my Rural Business management degree for what it was designed for.

CHAPTER THREE

I definitely didn't have all my ducks in a row as I grew up thinking they should always be. As a recovering perfectionist, even writing this book has been a challenge. Always thinking it's not quite good enough, but it is what it is and I believe its heaven commissioned, and who am I to not write it?

Now my daughter Hayley needs a chapter of her own! The chunk of love, who taught me love……

I cannot tell you how many times I have prayed that an instruction book came out with the placenta of "How to grow Hayley" because it feels like from the minute she was born my world has been rocked. It has been flipped over, turned inside out, flushed down the toilet, spun around on the teacups, and here I am looking and feeling like I have been dragged through a hedge backwards at times! I will never be the same again.

Where the heck was the training course for how to be a parent before you even conceive? because I think that more needs to be made of that. I wasn't prepared for what happened when I looked into the eyes of my darling daughter, because all through my pregnancy everyone, and I mean everyone, even the midwives had convinced me I was having a boy. We didn't find out at the 20-week scan, and I am glad I didn't else I wouldn't have had anything to be excited about with what ended up being a very rough pregnancy! More on that later!

Anyway, baby Hayley, a girl, was introduced to me by my darling mum, because she had come out so darn quick the midwife was busy making sure she didn't drop her! Then it struck me, I was a girl as well (cue music: dum dum dum) 24 years it took me to realise this, and I never ever wanted Hayley to be anything like me, or rather feel like me or act like me. I knew then I was in trouble!!!

From that moment on I didn't realise it, but my heart endeavoured me to take on the biggest challenge I would ever have to take on. That was to learn to love myself, for who I was warts and all. It was scary because when you become a mum you are responsible for this new human being. I had to keep it alive. I knew how to keep animals alive because there had been many a night, where I have been sat up tending to a weak or poorly lamb. I knew I had to feed it, keep it warm and hope it got better. That lamb however could be left with the sheep, and it was what it was by the morning.

This was not a lamb though, oh no! And who knew about purple crying! I would never believe a newborn baby could scream its little lungs out until it was purple, to the extent that neither Andrew nor I could do anything with her. Leaving her in the end to cry it out and hopefully fall asleep which is what she did. That was just the start of that one because Hayley developed this wonderful condition called reflux. This is where her milk would literally come back up, sometimes she would vomit, sometimes you just heard the bubble pop and then screaming. Such intense screaming which created as much pain in me as it did in her, because she was a part of me. My baby was in pain and like so many I was going to do everything in my power to get her fixed. No mother likes to see, hear or sense the pain within her child. And that is often linked to a deeper pain within herself, an unhealed soul wound more than what is going on in the child. When we parent from those unhealed wounds, it too can cause more damage to our children than we could imagine.

Let's face it, in this world pain is inevitable, and as is the case in the film Inside Out, you can't have happiness without its best friend sadness. Anger is there to drive us, not abuse anyone, disgust stops us eating poison, and fear, well fear is interesting because it has the same chemical reaction in the body as excitement. It depends if you have lived in a place of fear and uncertainty or love and compassion. Fear to me is the root to most of our problems, and when you are living in it, you don't see that it is more dangerous than anything.

Whenever I mention being stressed to people who I can see are pretty stressed, they will just about always say, "but I don't feel stressed". Stress comes from being afraid, not feeling safe and this can of course come from any point in our lives, before birth even. Fears can even be passed down through generations, as learnt behaviours.

I have noticed in Hayley how stressed she can become. She has all the outward physical signs which I recognise, not being able to go to sleep, wanting to watch more of her screen than engage with the world, certain ticks and things her body does which shows me she is afraid of something. Something has triggered her central nervous system to go into fight or flight, and if I ask her about it she won't have a clue. Yet I on the other hand often know exactly what has caused it, and will talk to her about it so she can learn to get to know her own body. If an adult doesn't point out to a child what is happening in a loving and honouring way, they will turn into adults who are living in stress having no clue that they are stressed. With no knowledge of how to alleviate the problem.

I want Hayley to be different and I will do all I can to make this happen, because I don't want her to become like I was. I have realised on my journey that I lived in a state of chronic stress which led to burn out on multiple occasions, sometimes taking months or years to recover. I have learned about Hayley through the challenges she has had, from school refusing to self-harming, from not wanting to go to school, to having to take her out and home educate her. I started assessing myself, and what happens when I get stressed. I am the best Neuro-coach to myself first! Once you start to see what your brain is thinking, and how your body is reacting to the thoughts through emotions, which is energy in motion, you can then start to work out how to stop your central nervous system going awol over every little situation, which is really not helpful as a parent.

Being in a state of constantly being triggered because your brain is deciding to spin you a heap of thoughts which are lies, is exhausting and one of the main reasons women struggle to function sometimes, just on a basic level, like keeping the house organised, or feeding the family cooked meals. Our brains can be so cram packed with unhelpful thoughts which are getting us nowhere, we struggle to be the mum we truly want to be.

We have learnt that pain and sadness is a bad thing and must be avoided at all costs, especially when your child is in pain. This is not good for the child and can completely trigger the mum to want it to stop. In Ireland they have a saying "they have sadness on them", rather than "I am sad" because it doesn't have to be part of who we are, it's just something that we can be going through and can be changed. It is a privilege to be able to have such complex emotions because if we didn't life would just be boring. But we have so many different emotions some of which we don't even realise we have!

CHAPTER FOUR

I have a book which lists lots of emotions that we as humans have, it is not just the few that we learn in school. I consider learning about our emotions to be so important to our family, that we have 4 posters on the wall next to the kitchen table, so that we the adults can learn new ways we can process them healthily. Not pushing them down and not pouring them out onto those we love. Which is sadly what ended up happening with Hayley from about the age of 4-8. I was her safe person and I had to completely sort my own reactions out to make sure Hayley could learn a new way of dealing with how she was feeling inside. You see every time I got angry with Hayley and shouted and screamed, I was inadvertently doing more and more damage to my beautiful girl and teaching her that this was the way to deal with her emotions. She then of course went about shouting, screaming and hitting me all the time. It's like the intensity of her reaction doubled compared to mine, and that's what I have witnessed happening generationally. Every generation since World War 2 has developed more and more mental and emotional problems. We don't have to look very far to find a child or adult who is struggling mentally.

The power of observation is amazing though and researching things and even learning to be present in situations, without these things I wouldn't know what I know now. Some people say I know too much, or I look into things too deeply, but that's what I love to do especially when it comes to Hayley and my fascination with her. Her whole-body health started when she had reflux which was causing physical pain, now I look back I can see exactly what happened. I took Hayley to a cranial therapist when she was three weeks old, she told me that because Hayley had come out like a rocket, she didn't uncoil herself properly meaning her spine was all twisted. She wanted to stay curled in a ball, not lie out flat on her back like the health visitor said she should, and the bones in her skull were slightly over lapping. Once it had been pointed out to me, I could see what she meant. The pressure in her little head must have been quite intense.

The cranial therapist uncurled her for me, and after a few weeks things improved a little, but we spent many a night sleeping sitting up together to help her tummy settle. There was still something going on, and what I didn't know then was about the effects of taking pain medication which was going through my breast milk and into my baby's tummy, which was probably causing the reflux, I didn't find out that one until Hayley was about 6.

Thankfully she is fine now, with no lasting tummy effects, they went once she was on bottled milk, unlike all my physical health conditions, which was the main reason of stopping feeding her in the first place. It was thought that if my hormones could return to normal than my pelvis would stop slopping around and I would not be in as much pain. Admittedly I did loose 3 stone stopping breast feeding, but no pain went away, and I still wasn't able to walk very far without crutches. To this day I still regret stopping feeding her myself, but we live and learn, and we do what we think is best at the time.

This was the first look into a fascination or rather obsession I now have on just how does the body work? How was it designed? How am I a physical, emotional, and spiritual being? What is my soul? What is my mind? What are my emotions? A big one, how is what I am feeling on the inside portrayed on the outside? How are my actions and words what I do and say every day, connected to the way I am feeling inside and the life I am choosing to create.

Hayley became fascinating to me; her perfect little body was like a clean sheet to start a new life literally. This baby knew nothing of how to exist on the outside of me. She has had to learn everything, from eating, pooping, walking, talking and who is her biggest role model? Me of course! And you are the biggest role model to the children you may have in your life. They don't even need to be your kids, I have nieces and nephews that I love having in our life, and I intentionally make sure that I am showing them a better way to think and feel about things, so that when they are grown up, they have the coping mechanisms I didn't have.

CHAPTER FIVE

The key I've discovered to becoming the woman, mum, wife, daughter, sister only ever seemed to exist in the movies, the one that seemed to have it all together and things worked out well for them. They could have the children, run a house, have a career, have a fantastic life and be the best role model to their children is, you must learn to love yourself, and in doing that realise you will never be perfect, because the films only ever give one side of the story most of the time. And guess what? You don't have to be perfect, because the world isn't going to be perfect any time soon, so we all fit right in. Perfectionism as I mentioned before is slowly killing us and preventing us living the lives God always intended for us.

Our families deserve the best version of us, heck we deserve the best version of us, not the half asleep, half drunk on anything but a good life, so busy we miss all the amazing things about being a mum, wife, sister, daughter version. Just today I held Hayley's hand walking into Tesco, and I thought I want to remember this moment forever because one day her hand won't be that small anymore. I often also stop and be thankful to my parents because one day things will change. So many of us are sleepwalking through life and the scary part is we don't even realise it. It is like the level of spiritual warfare has gotten so bad in our nation, we struggle being a mum, hating it at times because we can't measure up to the worlds standards of motherhood.

You know the mother that bounces back within weeks? That has an organised and tidy home? That has more than the one child in my case. This has been a hard one for me because we have only been able to have one, we don't ever feel like we are good enough and often can be found wondering what the heck am I going to do? How am I going to get through this? The world has gotten faster, more hi tech, more connected than ever. Yet the belief that we have to do everything on our own, is drilled into us from school, and is leaving us lonelier than ever.

The number of mums I see posting looking for friends breaks my actual heart. Where are the villagers around us helping us to bring up our children in this mad world? We need them, we need each other, we need the help of our parents if they are still here to do it.

One of the most powerful scriptures in the bible for me and the one I use the most is "We do not battle against flesh and blood, but against the rulers, authorities, powers of this dark world against the spiritual forces of evil in the heavenly realms." Ephesians 6:12-13. The biggest problem we face in the world today is that we don't believe that there are any invisible forces at work whether they are good or bad ones. Heck, we don't even believe there is a God who had to have created the world because it's far too complex for man to have even contemplated making it, or it just banged into existence. We are just very good at ruining the world, and I for one don't want my daughter to be sleep walking around, unaware that there is a divine plan for her life, and unless she decides to pursue it then she could end up in a whole heap of trouble.

To be honest, before I became a Christian and I knew about any of these things, Hayley ended up in a whole heap of physical mental and emotional trouble because of me, and doing things my way and not Gods. And because there is a spiritual enemy out there working against us. Once I figured out that as a believer in Jesus and as Hayleys mum that I could have spiritual authority over her, then things started to change for the better. Philippians 4: 6-7 says, "do not be anxious for anything, but in every situation, by prayer and petition with thanksgiving, present your requests to God. And the peace of God which transcends all understanding, will guard your hearts and your minds in Christ Jesus."

Every day I say to myself "how does anyone parent without Jesus, how does anyone do anything without Him?" Because I can honestly say for me that is what has changed everything in mine and my families' lives. I am not writing this book because it's a nice thing to do although it is. I am writing this book because I feel called to write it because in it contains information that I hope and pray will change many lives.

This is me, the good, the bad and the ugly, and the reason I share my heart with you is because I believe there is absolutely a more excellent way for us all to live. To get the best out of this life whilst we are here, not look back and be filled with regrets. It takes courage, it takes stamina, but if I can do it anyone can!

CHAPTER SIX

Nothing could have prepared me for what motherhood has done, no one ever warns you that when you have a child it is like your heart is walking around on the outside of you and that's weird. All your instincts are set to "I have to keep this child alive" and your body may never look or act the same again, sometimes in a good way and sometimes not.

Parenting a child, I now see as a woman, is the single most important job I will ever do, and although I will always love my daughter, I only have a short window of time where she needs me to do absolutely everything. Then one day she will need me less, maybe just for listening, hugs and cooking her food every now and again.

You see at 8 years old my daughter Hayley I can see is sailing towards the time where she really is capable to do things for herself and that's how it should be. The only thing I must worry about is if I am training her properly to go out into the world and be armed and dangerous to make the change that's so needed. I want to raise a girl who people will be a little bit scared of, one who will fight for what is right, one that will want to protect others, and will want to bring about change to make the world a better place. Basically, in this instance I am raising a miniature version of myself.

Proverbs 22:6 says, start children off on the right path, and when they are older, they will not leave it. The only thing is for a very long time I wasn't on the right path for various reasons. The main one being I had no idea there even was a right or wrong path. Now I know I am on the right path, it's taken a while and I have got a lot wrong however I am determined to rewrite our future, so I can model peace, love and joy to Hayley, so things will be a whole lot simpler for her. This is available for anyone if you are willing to run the race and put in the effort, which it takes to change a family's future direction.

This is my challenge now and has been since Hayley was born, to start creating a life that I am choosing, to help make our lives easier not harder. If you are in farming you may think that's impossible. Instead of having a life where I made things hard for myself. I was working hard physically, I was doing the hours and also doing things that were getting me nowhere. It bit me in the butt when it came to having Hayley because it was like my body was trying to divorce me, it was no longer on my side. I kind of always knew I would have a baby by the time I was 25, so after nearly 2 years, 15 months not really trying, 9 months trying I was crying every month by this point, our gorgeous girl arrived in March 2014.

For a farmer having a spring baby was wonderful because that's when the babies are born, but it was also our busiest time with lambing and calving. This particular year all the sheep had finished lambing before she was born, so my mum could be at the birth, to save my poor husband who would have probably found it difficult sitting through my labour alone. I was in so much pain that wasn't just labour pains. My mum had to make some decisions I couldn't make in labour, so that I didn't end up in the same position as her with me, which was an emergency C-section.

Then finally there she was, my beautiful baby girl. I was expecting her to be a boy because everyone told me she would be, and that was what farming families wanted right? A boy to take on the farm. As I held her in the hospital, I knew without a shadow of a doubt I was in trouble. You see being a girl in farming had not been easy for me, in fact at that time I had never realised just how women in farming are ostracized, how we are looked upon as being the weaker sex, useless unless we could lift 25kg bags of feed, sling a small ball of hay on our back, do a hard day's graft on not much sleep, raise the children, cook the dinners, do the paperwork and go out to work. Because farming isn't managing to put food on the table, which is ironic don't you think?

This is what I believed, that being a woman in a farming family was hard especially since I had just spent the last 4 months walking around on crutches. But holding that girl in my arms, suddenly I knew I needed to change everything for her, especially when it came to our family and our farming business. And if I manage to change a small bit of the world around me at the same time, then that would be a bonus. Of course, looking back I realised these things, because there in hospital I had just had a 36-hour labour, needing an epidural and narrowly avoiding a c section. Having such deep thoughts back then was not happening, but since then they have happened and I have done some serious thinking. My dad says this is dangerous, he doesn't like my "I have an idea face". Yet thinking outside of the normal box, has brought about some serious changes to just about every part of my life, it has been completely turned upside down for the better.

Just to clarify there is nothing wrong with being physically strong enough to lift heavy things as a woman or indeed be farming as a woman. I am still able to, which is miraculous considering the damage I had done to my body. However, if we believe that its only if we do those things the men in our life will respect us, and treat us as equals, we are wrong because all these things gained me was a lower back shot to shit, a pelvis that I thought was going to fall apart and a mind that was screaming at me, "you are not good enough because you can't walk".

Everything happens for a reason and through the strangest of events just after, I joined an amazing British skincare company in 2014, I discovered that my true super powers was in my brain, not in what I could do physically. Since having this revelation, I can now see that it is my beautiful mind and thoughts which decide what my daily decisions and actions are, which are worth millions to my farming family, and that's not just financially, but relationally and health wise as well. Purely because I now have more time, I am more organised, and I am not running my body into the ground physically, by not having enough sleep or having harmful eating habits due to using food to regulate my stress levels, made worse by the diet industry, I won't get started on that now it needs a book of its own.

You see women bring to the farming industry something which men can struggle with, especially after having children, this was what changed things for me. Until I had Hayley, I had a very hard heart towards things which would happen on the farm, things dying, having to use lots of medicines to keep things going, and not considering the environment around us hardly at all. We weren't being stewards of the land, we were just focusing on producing more food, which ended up being lower quality. The soil under my feet was as hard as my broken heart by the time I became a mum. Both of which have now begun to soften as I embrace life through the eyes of love rather than fear.

CHAPTER SEVEN

Pregnancy, the blessings and the curses. The first year of Hayley's life was nothing as I imagined it to be, I had visions of having a baby strapped to my back out checking the sheep, rolling sheep over to do their feet, lambing and all that I had done for the previous 15 years of my life as a shepherdess, but it would seem that this was not to be the case.

At around 20 weeks pregnant I did what I now deem to be a silly thing, but then it was just a normal thing. Because I wasn't ill, I was just pregnant of course, I could just carry on lifting and carrying and running about as normal. I laugh at my naivety now, what a wally I was! One day I caught a lamb between my knees because it had a sore on its nose, and I am a dab hand with the blue spray to help this little sore heal in double quick time. I am straddling this lamb and I feel the tiniest of twinges in my left thigh. Hardly anything, just a little niggle. I gave it a rub and carried on climbing over hurdles working with the sheep. That little niggle however developed into a big niggle very quickly and before I knew it, I was having to crawl up the stairs, and take my mobile to have a bath just in case I needed to call the fire brigade to get me, the beached whale out. Thank God that never happened! my darling husband did it instead, he was my knight in shining armour, or rather cow poop covered armour.

This was when I realised what a blessing it was to still be living in the annex next door to my mum and dad, because I honestly don't think I could have coped being here by myself all day moping about not being able to move, not being able to drive and not being able to do anything like I had been doing before. This was when all aspects of my health started to slide. And I realised I was in trouble.

It didn't take long for my midwife to diagnose Symphis Pubis Dysfunction (SPD) or for some reason they decided it needed a name change so is now called Pelvic Girdle Pain (PGP). This is a condition that effects 1 in 5 women in pregnancy, and I personally believe that is because we are not taught how to take care of our backs properly, or even how to take care of our bodies properly as women.

Particularly women in farming, which let's face it, is still a man's world physically. We can be constantly competing or trying to keep up with the physical work the boys do. Not taking a blind bit of notice of the fact that they don't have to grow or carry the babies!!!

I was even warned by a farmer once, he must have been in his 70s, whilst working in a shop that sold animal feeds. As I was throwing bags weighing 25kg into the back of his truck. He said, "You shouldn't be doing that dear, you will hurt your back, my wife used to be like you and when it came to her having children, it caused havoc to her back". 19-year-old me was too arrogant and too stupid to listen then of course. I just laughed it off, I probably gave him some jibe and forgot all about it. When I remembered it though, those words haunted me.

What came was a complete physical melt down, crutches by 24 weeks pregnant, nearly in a wheelchair by week 34. I couldn't drive for fear of getting stuck somewhere. I had to have chaperones and I am forever grateful to those beautiful friends and family of mine, who took time out in their day to drive me to appointments. I became a baby making machine who watched, Murder She Wrote and Poirot every afternoon, I was able to cook tea for the family just, and then I would play candy crush until 3.00am so I didn't have to be in bed with my husband for too long, because the pain was excruciating. We kept rolling together, 2 years later when his back was hurting, we changed the bed and mattress that's typical isn't it? anyway!

The strange thing was SPD/PGP is a condition where you can't just stay still because it makes it worse, and you can't move loads as it makes it worse. It's basically a nightmare and lots of trial and error of what you can and can't do before the pain is so bad it takes you days to recover. I went to a physio who made it worse because she had no real experience with this condition. I refused to take any pain relief because I didn't want anything going in my body whilst I was pregnant. I didn't even take paracetamol, managing the pain with hot baths and the right mix of sitting, standing, lying, kneeling, moving and pregnancy yoga which was the only night I ever really slept after a session.

But it was ok because I was cooking a baby, I told myself, which I had longed to have. Most women see a complete recovery 8 weeks after having the baby. It was all going to be ok, or so I thought. 8 weeks post pregnancy came and went, and I found myself sending my mum into different pharmacies to get my co-codomol, which helpfully says "don't take for any more than 3 days, because you can become addicted" because that's all that would dull the pain just enough so I could sort of get on with life. Apart from the days I had to get my mum to get me out of bed, and of course the days when I couldn't go anywhere because I couldn't carry a baby and walk on crutches.

I continued with my home pain remedy concoction of paracetamol, ibuprofen and co-codomal in the hope that one day it would all magically go away. Which of course it didn't, instead on Hayley's first Christmas my body went into full scale rebellion, I had nearly 20 ulcers in my mouth and I knew it was the pain meds. I went to the doctors to be told that I wasn't addicted to them because I wasn't taking over the stated dose, never mind the 3 days maximum warning on the box.

The doctor that day judged me so badly, she had 5 children and was a doctor, and here I was after one child, moaning about a bit of back ache. Now I know that I actually spiritually feel the judgements of others, and this has caused lots of damage to my soul. People don't even need to say anything, which is why I work so hard to not judge anyone by what I am seeing, or even hearing. But it's hard because humans are complex and we are sadly wired to judge, and this is a part of spiritual warfare I am grateful I have been able to discover, mainly so I can protect myself and have stronger spiritual boundaries. Matthew 7:5 says take the plank out of your own eye, and then you will see clearly to remove the speck from your brother's eye. Judging one another does more harm than good, and the doctor that day made me feel so bad I chose to never trust the NHS for this situation with my pelvis ever again.

There were dark days, I was in a pit of misery. I cried more than I ever had because I was grieving for the loss of everything that I had known to be true to that point. I felt like crap and knew I had to go cold turkey and come off the pills and jeez that wasn't fun, because nothing had changed from my pregnancy, and as for my mental health! Well, that was a mess. Being busy with a new baby, I hadn't even noticed the state of my own mental or emotional health. That is because I had never even known or considered that I had mental and emotional health. I was too strong for all that. (oh Leanne, you plonker!) I can't remember any lessons in school teaching me about how you think and feel has an effect on your life, because there wasn't any, the science just wasn't there, but now it is.

It wasn't until one day I stood to leave my house and I considered that I had to go down a road and cross over a dual carriage way to deliver some skincare products to a customer. That day I stood in my lounge and thought. "I am going to die if I cross that road. We are going to have a massive car accident, I won't be able to get Hayley out, and the car might set on fire, other people may run into us. We are going to die."

CHAPTER EIGHT

Now I had seen what happens when people have anxiety and panic attacks, which are invisible to other people, but they are very real to the one having them. If you allow it too, it takes over your life, and before you know it you can't leave your house by yourself. In fact, your life becomes all about the what ifs and your over imaginative brain starts to rule the roost. Get this, your brain sees it that when it creates these kinds of thought patterns it is protecting you. Our brain is always trying to keep us safe based on what has happened in our past, it then projects into our future through our decisions and actions. Our brain as helpful as it is, is still essentially based in the cave man days, thinking we have man eating animals running after us, yet for the majority of us this isn't true, but the reaction in the body is the same fight, flight or freeze. Our brain unless trained to do otherwise will recall, memories of situations and use them to stop us in our tracks or run for the hills. This is why if you ever want to do something different with your life, you often can't, you may make a start but if a thought creeps in it will stop you. This is also known as our comfort zone.

And what I saw back then in myself and what I see now in many people is that a brain that has not been disciplined or trained in any sort of way, to capture its own thoughts, slowly can end up ruining your life, your kids' lives, your partners lives and anyone else in your close friends and family because you are having a hard time being able to have the life you really want. I have seen many other dark days since those, but back then I didn't have any real hope of better days to come. Nothing that I could really believe in anyway, I wasn't a believer in anything other than myself, and now I know it was myself that got me into the state I was in.

Looking back, I did have something, I had this small quiet voice within me that would say to me daily, "you are going to get through this, and you will be healthier and happier than you ever were".

I now know that voice to be the small quiet voice of God leading me back to where I belonged in Him through Jesus. This was just the beginning of what was going to be the start of a whole new life, I just didn't know it.

Since becoming a neuro-coach and learning about the power of neuroscience and what happens in our brains automatically, without us even noticing 90 percent of the time. I can now see how I was in a place where I really didn't feel safe, because of my physical disabilities and when you think a thought like the one I mentioned above, your emotions kick into make sure that you stay home. In this case and essentially in most cases what kicked in was the emotion of fear. That fear is what I have slowly learnt to override over the years, using the power of Jesus because he doesn't give us a spirit of fear but of power, love and sound mind. 2 Timothy 1:7. I more than ever want a sound mind right now, just so I can be the mum I truly want to be.

Your mind is where your thoughts happen, biblically this is called the carnal mind. It tries protecting you by generating negative thoughts based on your past experiences, which we have let in unknowingly from childhood even before we are born. Once upon a time they may have once kept you safe, but now you don't need them because you're an adult and can think rationally, you can discern better what is right and wrong, and hopefully ask enough questions to get the right answers to have a safer life. The negative thoughts may have been spoken over you by adults inadvertently causing harm, or you have thought them about yourself. What ends up happening, is you have an invisible battle inside of yourself every single day. One part of you wants to do lots of fun and exciting things, be present with your kids, provide everything you want them to have, in my instance is a successful business as well, and the other is side of you is going NOOOOOOOOOO we can't do that because of …

Normally all the thought patterns that are stored in your sub conscious mind, are stuck to an emotional response in your body. This makes it even harder to win the battle of your mind. You see other people are living amazing lives and you wonder why you aren't, it's because of your belief system and how you think needs an upgrade, and many of us need healing on a deeper level as well, which can be a scary prospect in itself.

An Example

Someone has just said to you as a 4 year old "don't be so stupid' this was said to you your entire life and when it was first said to you, you thought it meant "you're stupid". At the time as a small child, you associated stupidity with not being perfect, so you didn't fit in, you weren't good enough just as you were, a 4-year-old, trying to learn how to live in the world. The emotions you may have felt were guilt, shame, and fear. Fear is what creates the response anger. For a little while you hear this said, "don't be so stupid" and you thought it meant you were stupid and the same feelings come back. Shame, guilt, fear. In the eyes of a child nothing is stupid to them, even the smallest of things can be gigantic to a small child. Yet us parents take that completely for granted.

One day though when you are a bit older the response that comes out is anger. Anger so powerful that you feel like you are the ruler of the world. Especially as a teenager, that anger however then starts stripping relationships with parents, siblings, grandparents, strip by strip. Anger suddenly has a stage, and it is going to keep coming out until it has done what it aims to do steal, kill and destroy family relationships. Leaving nothing but tatters, hard hearts and relationships that run on hatred, fear, control and manipulation. Not love, honour and peace.

You see, if you dear friend are a woman who's mind and thoughts run in a similar way, to what mine did. Its overly anxious, the thoughts are whirring around in there and you lose your temper daily with whoever you love the most.

From this moment on I want you to know, it is not your fault. It was never your fault, we have just never learnt about our mental and emotional health, and the power it has over our bodies if we let it control us. You see when our mind says something repeatedly over and over, let's take the "You're stupid" example again then to save energy your brain goes "oh this thought needs, to be automated and puts it into the sub-conscious, where it can run on autopilot", because it has been repeated. Science says 67 times is all we need to repeat something for it to really stick and become a thought pattern, that turns into a belief.

Our sub-conscious runs in the background doing useful things like telling our body to breathe, our heart to pump, stomach to digest, as well as helping us do all the tasks we need to do, all very important and we don't actually have to think about those things every day. This is how we can eventually drive a car without thinking about it, and brush our teeth on autopilot, if you try brushing your teeth with the other hand it's a different story entirely, its quite awkward. However, the brain does the same for other things in your life as well which aren't so helpful. I had a thought which kept me making my house untidy, so I used it as an excuse to procrastinate and not do more important things, that I wanted to do like write a book, spend time with friends those kinds of things. Because writing a book is something different, something new it might not be safe to do that. And inviting people over when the house is in a mess is a dangerous thing to do because it opens us up to being judged. This is what the sub conscious is saying behind the scenes to stop us from ever being able to do things out of our comfort zones. This for me has caused a lot of internal stress over the years.

CHAPTER NINE

Anger is powerful and dangerous. Anger doesn't just come out on others either, it can go the opposite way and you can swallow your anger, every single day of your life until it drains you of every ounce of energy you have, and it causes you stress you don't even know you are under. You end up run down all the time, tired, living a life that you don't want to live, and worse still if it carries on, your whole body's energy and immune system gets zapped, and you end up ill. It starts as a cold, but soon it becomes constant chest infections, urine infections, headaches, ulcers, chronic pain …….. (you fill in the dots) and then one day you can get told something you had never wanted to be told, and it could require far more treatment than some antibiotics or over the counter medications. If you are lucky enough to be able to have treatment and survive it.

I have done both, let my anger come out onto my family particularly my dad and Hayley, and I remember thinking when I was pregnant with Hayley that I didn't want to get stressed anymore, so I would choose not to get angry. Which wasn't healthy either because it just went inwards.

For me it never got to the stage of being told I had a terminal illness, and I hope that by sharing the things in this book that I have that you never get to that stage either and you will learn to start listening to your body, and loving yourself. But I did lose the ability to move and walk around properly. I thought I would never walk long distances again without crutches. You might ask what did you do with your anger then Leanne? Well, I did both things that I have just described, a whole lot came out of me onto other people including Hayley when she got to around 18 months. And a whole lot went inwards causing the energy to be sucked from me, making me gain weight and to be in a constant state of chronic stress, which I am still learning to deal with now.

You see, yes, I did injure myself catching that sheep one day whilst I was pregnant, but really and truly that was the least of my problems. What happened to my body was a combination of things which had been building up all through my life, traumas I had collected up and not known what to do with them which is why recovery has been so long, 10 years as in writing this part of the book. I had a quad bike accident at 14, I held mental and emotional trauma in my body, to make it worse I held other people's traumas in my body, and it was exhausting. I had a sensitivity to the needs of others just being in the room with them and I never even knew it. You could say I was always destined to be empathetic, to be so sensitive I could tell there was something going on within the bodies of people just standing next to them, and when those people are your family, it becomes difficult to have good boundaries, because these are the people you love and have loved you.

CHAPTER TEN

Being in a farming family caused huge amounts of these mental and emotional traumas. Since I have been born in the 90s everything has been changing in farming. The government stopped paying us to produce food, they want us to grow trees or wild bird food instead. We have legislation and red tape around all sorts of things for animal welfare and the safety of humans. Diseases like BSE, Foot and mouth TB, bird flu seem to be rife, and outbreaks have been poorly managed. I was 13 when foot and mouth happened and I was so afraid I had to move out, I just couldn't bare the thought of bringing back something to our animals from school. These things put immense pressure on my parents and essentially on my brother and I as well.

Where once farmers were unsung heroes, it seems we are now the scape goats for everything that goes wrong from not creating enough CO_2 to put into coke and beer cans when we stopped buying artificial fertiliser, because the price had shot up and we were in the middle of a drought. To our cows causing so much methane with their farting which is actually burping that they must be the issue and are causing climate change. Yet when all planes were grounded and cars stopped during Covid lockdowns the air cleared up, and as far as I can see cows didn't stop burping. We apparently are causing all the water pollution, yet private water companies are discharging raw sewage all the time and getting away with it. Who is really at fault here?

Growing up on a beef and lamb farm has been hell at times, and the echo's of my parents voices telling me to not come home farming, but to go and do something else is ringing in my ears even more so. Yet it's like my heart is pushing me forward all of the time, despite the struggles, despite the feeling of not being wanted by the UK government and consumers even, the little quiet voice I mentioned before is still there willing me on. Not just for my sake but for the sake of lots of others as well. Because farmers are important to this country, and even to the world. We have knowledge that far surpasses that of people who just learn farming from text books, or as they go.

Farming has been observed for generations in my family, and it's those observations that run deep, they run so deep it's taken me over 30 years to realise I do the things I do, I see things I see, and I know the things I know. The skills and the knowledge that I and countless other generational farmers have far surpasses the big wigs who think they know it all.

But when truth be told and the shit hits the fan and we are stranded on an over populated island in the middle of nowhere unable to feed the nation. It'll be us that are turned to for the solutions, and we that is all generational farmers will do what has been built into us to do and that's supply your children and families with food. If there are no farmers, there is no food!

The sooner we wake up to this fact, and stop pretending that fake food grown or made in a laboratory is going to save us the better, because it's not going to save us it's going to make us sick.

CHAPTER ELEVEN

Setting Boundaries. I was never very good at setting boundaries, it turns out this is challenging when you have ADHD which I have diagnosed myself with using the plethora of information on the internet. I have struggled regulating my emotions, which leads to unhealthy behaviours like overeating and used to be over drinking, I have struggled to say no to things, to cram too many things in the diary and then feel stressed out. Before being a mum I used to be quite organised, but a complete control freak with everything, which meant I was stressed out all the time really wanting everything to be controlled. I didn't notice any real issues until I became a mum and then things just seemed to go AWOL. Which is the case for many women it seems.

The truth is before I became a mum I had no real time or emotional boundaries of any sort. I kind of just went along with things until I got poorly. Many farming families don't have any boundaries, they will work from dawn until dusk 7 days a week, they find it hard to take quality time out with family. They allow others to control them and are not able to make their own decisions, without being made to feel guilty about wanting to do things differently. Many farming families I know have split up because of this, and every day I am reading posts from within the farming communities where women are literally at the end of their tether not knowing what to do for the best, exhausted with the constant pressures of running a family farm.

For a long time, I believed that unless I was doing lots of hours of paid work then I wasn't good enough for anything else. My worth was well and truly in my work, yet now I know my worth is more than just working my butt off all the time. Its listening to someone who is struggling, its helping people solve problems, I love solving problems especially business-related ones. But more than anything my worth is in sharing my experiences with others because there is power in a testimony and once you realise all the struggles you have had to endure can actually be turned to good and to help others, then nothing else really matters.

Since realising I had suffered severe burnout I have discovered about boundaries and have been working on putting them in place. This has been one of the keys to be able to spend more time doing things that I enjoy and because of it I have more energy, this was key for when we decided to home educate Hayley. When I decided to do that, I had to say I wasn't going to be able to help so much on the farm. She had to become my priority, not the cows or sheep which looking back took priority in my lifetime. The farm always came first it felt like. I was left feeling like I had to fend for myself, never ask for help, work stupidly long hours and expect my body to just keep on going. Also, with home educating it took a whole life change, and until I worked out how we needed to spend our time which took a couple of years of doing. I also had my Tropic business which had to go on the back burner.

I wanted to do it all, be a mum, housewife, business owner. I wanted to spend time with friends, go on holidays, but because I was in so much pain all the time, my motherhood dreams were dashed. Just this week I found myself wishing that I had sorted out my life, which was coming from harbouring so much pain before becoming a mum, it would have been so much easier with far less pressure. Because let's face it I didn't want to mess my kid up so badly she needs a lifetime of therapy at the end of it. Yet that's what would have happened if I didn't take a long hard look at myself and realise, I had the power to change things for her. I accepted that my behaviour up to Hayley being aged 4 needed to change, because I was causing her emotional harm.

Then when we also lost my beautiful mother-in-law, this sent Hayley into a real mental and emotional spin. All of a sudden, she had no boundaries either, and was like a wild beast most of the time. She was so angry and had internalised my pain along with the pain of losing her granny. Many think that children don't know about these things, that they are resilient and don't need things explained to them.

This is a complete lie, because no matter what age a child is even before birth, they sense things, and know things on a deeper level. I have seen this in Hayley, it is like she knows what I am thinking, she knows when I am having a tough time and instead of pretending like I am fine and lying to her, I have started to tell her if I am angry or upset or if I have just woken up in a bad mood.

This helps her to create boundaries from me, I am teaching her that she doesn't have to take on other peoples negative energy. That she gets to choose to stay angry at someone or let it go if they are just having a bad day. But also stick up for herself when something has been said that is out of order. In the past she has been called names by other children, like they do children are very honest and we see it as cruel, but the world needs the honesty and that's a hard pill to swallow. I tend to just ask her is that true what that child has said to her. She will often say no, then I ask her what can she think about herself instead? We all get to choose what we think about ourselves, and we can choose to reject that negative words of others right from when they throw them at us.

As I write this there is a part of me that just wishes I knew these things before becoming a mum, what I know now about mental and emotional health, about thought patterns and negative energy. But I didn't and that's ok. I cannot keep condemning myself with my past mistakes. I can however work towards creating a better future for us and our children by having good boundaries, to protect my time, my energy and essentially my health, and you can too.

I want our lives to be thriving not just surviving, I want Hayley to know that she has a choice in life, to choose what she wants to believe about herself, and even about the world. I want her to know the truth and live within that truth about who she is and who God has created her to be.

In the quest to helping Hayley to be like this, I have ended up doing the same for myself, and it feels pretty amazing to know that potentially the last 5 generations of mental, emotional and physical pain, which has been handed down through our farming family. Through observing and learning behaviours of others has stopped because I stopped it. And this is a true mother's power to step in and say, "no more".

There is nothing more powerful on earth than the love that a mother has for her children, or in my case my daughter. I have found I would move heaven and earth for her if I could, and it is this love and deep desire for things to be different that continues to drive me on my path to wholeness. To be healthier in the future than I was in the past despite getting older. To be pain free and to not be needing medications for things because I have taken care of my body from now on. It's never too late, but it can be hard if you just don't know what steps to take next. That is where I can come in to help you work out what it is you need to do to get on the right tracks again.

CHAPTER TWELVE

Making babies is meant to be easy isn't it? Did you ever watch that film Look Who's Talking in the 90s, it had John Travolta in it and a baby who had a grown-up voice. At the beginning it showed the egg being fertilised by sperm and I think I grew up thinking that looked easy. That it all just happens with some sort of magic.

But to be honest, the making of the baby wasn't the easiest either. It wasn't one of those wonderful experiences of thinking about a baby and then conceiving, nope, it took us at least 9 months of actively trying, but I had been off the pill for nearly 2 years and secretly hoped I would just find myself pregnant one day. I remember the month before I conceived Hayley, I was sat in a tractor wrapping silage bales, as you do! And I was on the phone to my friend Alex bawling my eyes out, because I had come on my period again. I had been one of those women who believed my period was a curse in the first place, so I did not want to see it month in and month out, when all I wanted was a baby for goodness sake!

This and worst still, I know is the reality for so many women today, and there isn't a day that goes by that I don't count my lucky blessings we have one. Because baby number 2 as of writing this book hasn't decided to make an appearance yet either, after nearly 8 years of trying. Now I wasn't really planning to write about this experience because it is still a little raw and painful for me. But for the want in my heart of helping you see that just because some things don't turn out as we want them to turn out, it doesn't mean they are always wrong or that we are on the wrong track.

Now it has been our personal choice not to have any investigations done regarding this situation, that is because I have learnt an awful lot about hormones whilst on my journey of learning to love myself, and I am just not willing to put myself through it.

Anyone who decides to go through with the help of IVF or what other amazing way they can fertilise eggs and put them in wombs, I commend you. And for those of you who haven't been able to carry the child yourself, but have put your heart out there that little bit further, and decided to raise a child from another mother, you have my utmost respect.

I am blessed to have other beautiful children in my life who I get to sow time and energy into. My nieces and nephews, my friends' children, and girls mainly I work with through local church outreach projects. And I have come to terms with the fact that we were only supposed to have one and that is ok. It has come with its fears, but it has also come with many blessings. I am not sure I would have coped on my own healing journey with more than one, especially on big crash days where I don't get out of bed.

You see no matter who we are, whether we have children or not, there is a plan for our lives. There is a plan so big that our tiny little minds can't comprehend it. I know this deep in my heart because if I didn't know it, I wouldn't be sat here writing this book at 1.30 in the morning. You see science has now proven that we are 99% identical to each other, but the 1% we are completely different and if we don't ever truly discover what it is that makes us different, we will take it to our graves, and it will never do what its intended to do and bless other people, with our gifts and unique special sauce.

You see I now realise what I do is my 1%. I have a passion to see farming families thrive, in fact I have a passion to see all families thrive. I have been given the gift of speaking into the lives of others, whether through social media or in person. I have been gifted with a brain that works quickly at solving a problem, I love to solve problems, my own and others. I have also been gifted with vast amounts of knowledge about all sorts of things from farming, to parenting in love, to neuroscience, to selling skincare, to becoming healthy from the inside out.
This is before I even get into the spiritual gifts that I have of prophesy, teaching, evangelist, apostle and pastor. That's all I will say on those, but I can honestly say that the God I know who sent Jesus His son to rescue me wants us to have abundantly more in life than we may currently have, because I am living proof of it.

What I know is what I know, and unless I share it like I am now, it does nothing. It doesn't even have to be big things that we feel called to do, because it's in the small things that we can make the greatest difference. Like inviting a friend for coffee, because she has been on your heart, and you want to check in on her. If you aren't aware and sensitive to the needs of others because you have so much going on in your own head, you can never be truly present.

Just like I mentioned with me holding Hayleys hand, if I hadn't become present, rather than being stuck in the past or racing too far ahead into the future, I would miss some of the most precious moments of our lives. This was especially so as after 2 years in school we decided to home educate Hayley, and it's been the best thing ever for her and I, and for all of the family. If I hadn't learnt to coach myself though, keep moving forward even when it's been really hard and I have been full of doubt, if I hadn't kept releasing the suppressed pain, the soul clutter I had gathered up, rewiring my thought processes through Neuro-coaching then there is no way I could be here saying I am glad I made that decision.

We were never taught in school that within every newborn baby there is a blueprint to life waiting to be unveiled. Take learning to walk, talk or even before that learning to breathe, feed and poop. Have you ever stopped to think what is it that makes this child want to get on with life and live it? What is driving it to fall over and get back up? Why is that child so hell bent on climbing up on the windowsill when it's a 2 foot drop off the sofa when it lands headfirst.

It is because as babies and small children we are the most connected to the plan than we will ever be, because we don't have the sense of fear we can have in our teens, and into adult hood which can be made worse if brought up in a family not sensitive to your needs because they have so much fear. But somewhere around the age of going to school I believe, things shift, and we go from being driven divinely by the invisible force that makes us who we are, and we start being told what it is we need to learn.

If you ask Hayley why she didn't like school she will say "because they stopped us being able to play so much, we had to sit down and do work that I found hard". She found it hard I later found out because her little brain couldn't comprehend everything that she was required to learn whilst being in survival mode, trying to recover from a mother who had struggled mentally and emotionally from just before she was born, to then going through the grief process when her gran went home to heaven. Hayley had what is known as an emotional delay, which kicked in aged 4. It meant she was still displaying the same negative behaviour patterns right up until she was 8. This is what can happen to children, and it's what can have happened to us as well.

At school we learn that everything we ever do in life must come from someone else. That we aren't good enough to have our own ideas, that it is not good enough for us to be creative beings and sit for hours staring at a blank canvas wondering what to paint. That dancing and physical movement and acting is not a good way to make money and we should get a "proper" job. Instead, the very things we are learning, which are all important tools of course, I wouldn't be writing this without English, are the very things that put out our fires, stop us dreaming and stop us getting back up again because we believe that someone else knows better than us, and if we can't hit their standard then we aren't good enough for anything.

CHAPTER THIRTEEN

I believe here in the UK we are just starting to see how far this Who am I? epidemic is going to go, and it is going to be far greater than Covid. So many of us suffer with some form of mental health blips we shall call them, because they do not have to take over your entire life, I have plenty of evidence to prove that. I was a prime example of living the deemed to be normal life, I have a supportive family, I was working hard ridiculously long hours, I was earning my own money enough to do what I needed and wanted to do, but not enough to make any big changes in the world. That was ok for a time. But my focus was wrong, I was doing all these things to be a so-called normal person but who was I being?

I was a work hard play harder girl, filled with so much pain that I had collected up like each one of us does because we are human. For generations now it's been the belief that we must not show any weakness, because weakness is bad and now we are starting to reap the repercussions of this belief system here in the UK.

We are so disconnected from ourselves, our emotions and what we are thinking all the time and its causing major issues in us and in our children. We don't know how to be, because we have based everything around what we do. It is no one's fault that we have this soul clutter and that it is causing more and more pain as it goes down the generations.

Unless that is, you discover you have problems, and you choose to do nothing about it to get them solved. My soul clutter in my teens liked to drink, it liked to be numbed out most weekends to the point of oblivion. As for eating, yep, my soul needed and still needs and uses food to stop my emotions from rising to the surface, to keep me "stable". But my soul needed to be cleared out, and this for me has happened in multiple ways. I believe it mainly happened when I asked Jesus into my life to sort my crap out, to bring me divine healing. He has given me the people and all the steps that I have needed to do to get a real breakthrough in my physical health.

I found practical people like physiotherapists, cranial therapists, chiropractors. I talked to friends, accepted prayer from others. Being part of online groups of women who were a bit further ahead than me in life helped me through. Yet the greatest thing I have been blessed to discover is the ability to coach myself through Dr Shannon Irvine and her SINC Neuro-coaching programme. This is the science to the words in the bible to hold every thought captive. I learnt to write out my thoughts, all of them especially the ugly ones, the ones you can't believe you even think, and then I love to burn them so no one else must see or hear the contents of my mind ever.

This means when I spot the thought lurking there in my mind I can bring that thing out into the light, and it will no longer have any power over me. Once we start to see our negative thought patterns and the effects they have on our lives then that's where we start to see magic happen. When you change your thought patterns you change your future. Which is why I went on to train to be a Neuro-coach, and I still have my own Neuro-coaches that help coach me.

One of my greatest superpowers is to know exactly when and why I have been triggered by a situation, I know when my body is going into fight or flight or rather not coming out of the fight or flight reaction. I have gotten so sensitive to my own mind (thoughts, will and emotions), that if I need a sleep in the middle of the day, I know it's because my body needs it normally its fighting off an infection, or is exhausted from physical pain, or I just haven't been sleeping properly. I know what I am thinking when I am getting very stressed out about something, I notice my bodies reactions. I can label my emotions whilst they are happening. This has then helped me to help Hayley do exactly the same, in fact she will do it better than me because I am helping her to read her body, to tune into her thoughts and realise that she is in control of her mind and what she chooses to think or to reject.

There are now so many contributing factors that prevent us from ever truly discovering who we really are and what we are here for, and how a human even works it seems. So many of us are following the ideals of others, wanting to be like them so we have their lives instead of just discovering the best version of our own.

There are so many voices out there, do this and get this result, do that, and get that result but still within every single human being on this planet there is a small quiet voice inside. The one you don't hear very often because the world is too noisy, and you're trying your absolute best to drown out the noise of the voices in your head. I dread to think how many voices I used to have in my head before I started this journey, so much wasted energy and time, thinking things I didn't need to think.

Those voices I realised needed to be quietened which has taken some time, but it's happening and I am living in a different way. I see myself kinder, I treat myself kinder and I choose to think from a place of love rather than fear. I am more at peace now than I ever was, and the biggest thing I have noticed is that I have so much more energy. I have done nothing else to help with my energy levels, I haven't changed my diet, I haven't started some exercise regime that I have stuck to.

Nope, the only difference I have made to my life as of writing this is to get rid of the negative thought patterns I was having. And to rewire them with thoughts that are helping me live the life I have desired to have and have designed to be able to enjoy, rather than miss out because of feeling overwhelmed by everything that my brain was thinking about.

CHAPTER FOURTEEN

One day I took a pen and paper, I set a timer for 20 minutes and I wrote out every thought that came into my mind. It was the biggest load of crap you have ever seen, and I proceeded to burn it for fear someone would think I was insane. That is how bad it was, some of the thoughts I couldn't even write. But that day as I sat in our car, in a field at the top of our lane, I had a glimpse into the chaos that was my thought life and I thought, "I need to clear this out", it is exhausting having all this rubbish in there that has no good influence in my life at all. This is why I would get so tired all the time, and why I just couldn't do all things I needed and wanted to do every day. I have slowed my thought life down, I have created new thinking patterns to serve me and my family, and I have come up with lots of creative ideas for our farm business. The clarity of what I need to do for my next steps is unreal and something I never knew was even possible before.

Let's go back to the small quiet voice within, I believe and have experienced the small quiet voice within. The one that says something that you just dare to believe will happen. I had this with my injury whilst pregnant. The people around me who saw a heavily pregnant women on crutches had nothing but the worst things to say. "You could be on them forever", "you might need a new hip by the time you are 30", "how are you going to look after the baby?" All these seemingly harmless things, people just trying to help make me feel better, I guess.

I could have believed them and in the darkest of times I probably did. But there was this other voice, that just gave me faith that this wasn't the end, that this was only just the beginning, and I was going to get better, and I am. I can jump on a trampoline, run and ride a horse again, all things at one point I wasn't sure would happen. It took over 2 years to ditch the crutches, but I did it. All because I dared to believe the small voice, not the loud ones that didn't want me to have a pain free life.

The small voice I decided needed to become louder, I needed to hear this voice it was the one that I really wanted to believe, because if it was true I was going to get better and I wasn't just going to get better physically but spiritually, emotionally and mentally as well.

I believe the small voice knew what was best for me. It is this voice I believe is the one that gets a baby to take those first steps, that makes them want to talk and express themselves, and is the one that will guide you for your entire life if the world around you hasn't already drowned it out. To me this voice is divine and comes from the creator Himself who is creating for me an abundantly blessed life, the good life.

It is this quiet voice that is continuing to guide me in all situations I come up against daily. I have learnt to tune into it because I really want to live in a way that not only brings a change to my family's life but to the lives of others as well. If I stayed stuck in my own faulty thought patterns, I wouldn't be able to help anyone, because let's be honest back in 2014 I was struggling to help myself. Ok we haven't had a second child, I haven't gotten to complete physical healing just yet, but I am taking steps every day to get there. I have had so many answers to prayers from my granny being healed of mental health problems, to seeing our farming business to start thriving. But I have a lot of unanswered prayers as well, or the ones I have to wait for answers for.

When I first started writing this book, I was in a great place physically, writing this now I have gained weight and am not as mobile again and I have had to have a lot of treatment with my chiropractor, to undo 20 year's worth of damage.

Its like I have had to go back a little way to be able to come forward again. I have to wait, and I am ok now with waiting. I have got good at being more patient most of the time. And while I wait, I choose to do the other bits and pieces in my life that all adds up to the great life plan I have.

These include but are not restricted to, washing clothes, keeping the house clean, feeding our family, home educating Hayley, having fun, spending time with friends, thinking up ways I can express myself in the world, writing a book, collecting some more animals, running the farm in a way that serves us as a family. And, starting my own coaching business to help others to improve their health and their farming business as well. Because when we have learnt things through our own life lessons, we can share them with others to help them as well.

Just because we don't always get our own way in life, or rather it doesn't always go the way we think it should. This doesn't always mean that we should sit and wait for life to be over or do us over. Nope, in the disappointments that will always happen we must choose to use it to our advantage, learn a new lesson, open our hearts to new possibilities, learn to dream again and stop taking the precious time we have on this Earth for granted.

Time is the precious commodity that none of us seem to have just the "I am so busy" syndrome, yet we shall never get back this very moment. We are older today than we were yesterday and tomorrow we have no idea if we will see it. So, take courage in the fact that there is a plan for us, it can just take a little while to be able to see it but once you do you will never want to go back.

CHAPTER FIFTEEN

When you marry your best friend...I have shared about Hayley, it seems only right to share about my husband Andrew as well. As of April 2024 we knew each other 22 years!! We first met when I was 13 and he was 21, we worked together on the same farm. Although it is possible, I met him when I was 3 because my gran used to get her hair done next door to his mum and dads house, so I used to ask to go over and play.

We didn't become an official couple until 2010 when I was 21 after he had spent 5 winters in New Zealand. Being friends, I always went to say goodbye to him before he went but this time I didn't. He started writing me weird messages about missing me and promising to treat me like a princess. I will admit I was a bit like, "is he drunk at this very moment"? What is this random stuff he is saying, considering I had been one of the "lads" the driver to the pub for so long it was weird.

Anyway, I told him if he was being serious, he better take me out on a date, so he did and now we go to the same pub every year to celebrate, apart from 2020 of course, that year was kind of a write off for everyone.

That first date was funny, because we went from being friends to becoming more than friends but looking back, I feel like it was all set up anyway. Andrews mum even said to one of his sisters when I was 19 that we would get married, which I laughed at, but we actually did 4 years later. This was one of the first prophecy's I have had spoken over me and actually happen.

I always knew I would get married by the time I was 25 and I did, it was like a heart knowing. I won't say that I had a bit of a disastrous previous relationship history because, I am actually still friends with some of the lads I went out with before Andrew and I got married, but there were a few situations that I should just never have put myself in.

I was a rebel through my teens, I put my parents through hell let's say, the chances are you will know exactly what I mean so we will leave that one there.

I do count myself blessed to have married Andrew because he is the exact opposite to me, I guess that's where the other half saying comes from.

Where I am always flying around moving from one idea to the next the entrepreneurial spirit coming out in me, and my mouth tries to move at the same speed as my ADHD brain. Andrew often has an idea and sticks to it, willing to give things a go even if they don't work out the first time. The perfectionist in me however can struggle with trying new things out of fear of getting it wrong, but I am starting to push past the fear. I also used to have a very fiery temper and was the girl who everyone nicked named Lennox Lewis's sister because I would basically get drunk and start throwing my fists around. This is not something I am proud of now, but in the context of this book I feel it necessary to paint a good picture of the person I was before I became the person I am today.

I didn't just get angry when drunk either, often getting angry with my parents for what I look back and see as being nothing that was their fault. They like so many other parents could only do what they knew was best for me at the time. They did not have a clue why I was harbouring such anger deep inside, because I didn't know why I was harbouring it until recently.

We have so much more science and evidence which is helping us bring up our children differently now, the internet being a huge source of information that in the 90s wasn't there. Letting go of the past has been the most amazing part of my journey so far, being able to revisit things for the benefit of helping others but not being emotionally triggered any more, this is what happens when your soul wounds are healed, and you can use your story to connect with others on a deeper level to bring them breakthrough in their life. It really is pretty cool and one of the greatest discoveries I have had.

Andrew and I are also best friends and this I feel has been the key to our relationship, there really are no skeletons to jump out of the cupboard, because we kind of knew all the skeletons whilst they were happening.

I always thought it was mumbo jumbo about marriage never really taking it seriously, but as I see the marriages of others around us be nothing like ours, we really do honestly like each other even in public. I often take a moment to honour how truly blessed we are to have each other. It is a divine connection that I couldn't have created myself. Don't get me wrong here there are still those times that we have disagreements, but they are never in malice towards each other. Its normally me getting annoyed because Andrew likes to think things over more than I do. I just go ahead and do them. Or when I have been completely triggered by something I take it out on him, and that's what happens when you have a neurotypical person married to a neurodiverse person.

Does this mean we never fall out? Of course not, because there are times when things just bubble to the surface, and they are better out than in. But we know when to say sorry, we can humble ourselves enough to admit when we are wrong, and we can chat it out and often come up with a better solution to the problem than what we were doing before.

This is because the main thing, or should I say person we fall out about the most is Hayley. I hold my hands up in honour to any mother or father going it alone. I can honestly say I couldn't do it, and I think this is my many driving forces of making sure that both Andrew and I feel honoured in our marriage. His love language is quality time, so we make that time for us to be together even if it is just watching a film. My love language is acts of service of which he does well every day, he will often do the washing, and he will also do the dish washer just little things that I prefer him doing than getting me presents.

In our family it is all about teamwork, not about who is working the hardest or earning the most money. It should never be about who is lording it over who either, the whole situation between men and women that has gone over the generations in my eyes is utter rubbish and we have been fed the lie that women "should be seen and not heard" and quite frankly the women need to be heard.

She is a helper to the man. He needs her to complete the other half of him. Does that mean we should be in abusive relationships whether physical, verbal or sexual of course not, but it does mean that when we start seeing our marriages or any relationships as team work rather than, "I am the leader and you should bow to me", we will find that everything else becomes easier.

Human beings aren't designed to be alone, although we can end up alone because of the damage that has been done to our souls is so deep. We want to curl up and not allow anyone to see us, touch us, or help us. Loneliness is probably one of the biggest life suckers on this planet, because you can be surrounded by people and still feel lonely. I always felt like the black sheep in my family, what are you supposed to do then?

I will tell you what I did, I made sure that every single moment of my days was taken up by something that didn't make me have to address how I was truly feeling inside. Through my teens and into my 20s I worked my ass off, because I needed to make sure I was so exhausted I didn't have time to think about feeling lonely. I worked hard and partied harder, stopping only when my body had had enough, I would get poorly or throw my back out. This worked for me until like you have already read, I found myself physically incapable of walking unaided for a long time.

Then all of a sudden, the loneliness was real, and Murder She Wrote, and endless games of Candy Crush really weren't doing anything to help. Throw in a baby on the top and you have yourself a walking disaster zone waiting to happen. And poor Andrew just kept going for us, he works for us, he goes to bed early for us so he can get up early, he listens to both Hayley and I when we need him to, even in the middle of the night when Hayley and I are having a blazing row.

I must have been a complete nightmare to live with for several years after having Hayley, I can see it now and I probably treated him like utter crap, because I was afraid. I was afraid of what was happening, and I was afraid of what was going to happen.

The one thing a mother wants more than to have a baby is to be able to support that baby, and child as best as they can. But for the first few years of Hayley's life that wasn't the case, and Andrew took the brunt of my feelings of inadequacies and still does when I am going through a hard time.

And if he ever reads this, I want to say thank you Andrew for sticking with me in my melt downs and being the constant that I have needed in this roller-coaster we call life.

CHAPTER SIXTEEN

What we aren't told about parenting. Oh how I wish I had gone on this journey before becoming a parent, but it didn't happen that way, and often I have felt completely powerless when it came to the tough stuff of parenting like keeping a child alive, not letting her get sick, or worse still disciplining her so she could grow up to be a fully rounded human being, capable of doing anything she set her mind to and she felt called to do. This has been especially challenging because she is an only child. Then there is a guilt around not spoiling her too much, and making sure she feels loved and accepted but not responsible for her parents happiness all the time.

There is nowhere in a book that says, becoming a parent is the easiest things you will ever do. If you don't have children yet, then I have just prepared you! Parenting to me can be defined as this: The ability to create a human being from 2 broken souls, because that is what the world deems as the right thing to do. You don't need a licence to parent yet you need a licence to get married, drive a car, own a gun, be a doctor almost all other things in life needs a qualification except parenting. So where does that leave us? Running around like a headless bloody chicken, spinning as many plates as we can muster, hoping that we don't forget to feed the child in the frenzy. I was so glad when Hayley was able to say, "I am hungry mummy". I was one step closer to it being easier to keep her alive.

Something else I would have liked to know before becoming a parent is that I am able to have all my inner wounds healed, if I am willing to face them head on rather than stuff them down and hope they disappear. Then go about the business of rewiring my belief system and thoughts from a place of wanting a better future, rather than from my experiences from the past. If we don't stop it our pasts will keep projecting into the future, because children learn off their parents, so every generation can get worse until someone stops it.

I wish I had seen a councillor before being a parent rather than whilst being a parent, even though I know full well it was having Hayley in the first place that forced me to sort my shit out. And it would have helped me have a better relationship with my dad which I now thankfully have. Up until becoming a mum I wasn't high on my own list of priorities, now I am a mum I discovered I needed to be at the top of that list of priorities, so I could do all the things I want to do as a mum. Learning to love myself has been the greatest gift I've been given. Biblically God commands us to love your neighbour as yourself, yet how can you love your neighbour if you don't love yourself? And how do you love yourself without being selfish all the time? It's took a while to work through but I got there in the end and I truly love the person who I have become now, and that is regardless of what I look like, which has been a hang up my entire life.

In the last 8 years I have put my big girl pants on and started to unravel, with the help of others, the mess that was my mind, soul and body. It has been one of the hardest yet most fulfilling things I have ever done. It would have however been easier to do when I wasn't trying to parent as well. But hey here I am, and every day I am a step closer to feeling like super mum, rather than holy crap how am I going to survive this mum. I would even go as far as saying that it is having Hayley that keeps me on the track to discover who I really am, and who I can be once I have let go of the past, I can choose to live in the present and dream of our future.

An interesting fact I have discovered as well which I needed to be a parent for is that your children can mirror you, and of course they won't just mirror the good bits. Oh no, I remember the day Hayley and I were in a battle of wills, with each other she was aged 3 and I was aged 29 acting like a 3-year-old. I was like I don't like this one bit, why is she being like this? It was a little while later when I was thinking about it, that I realised I didn't like it because I didn't like that she was showing me my faults. She was copying my behaviour, it's a bitter pill to swallow sometimes but I have come to accept that if there is something I don't like about Hayleys behaviour, the chances are she has learnt it from someone, and that someone has a bigger chance of being me than her dad because she is with me 24 hours a day.

My way of dealing with anything was to get angry about it, shout about it, stomp around, slam doors and guess what, my gorgeous girl does the same even now, I have managed to address my anger issues and I am blessed to be able to help her with hers. I have more patience; I know when I am getting angry so I can warn Hayley before I fully get there. My weaknesses are still put to the test when something happens to Hayley and she responds in anger. I however manage most of the time to not completely lose it, even in public. I have gotten it down to a fine art I feel personally. My friend Laura would testify that after it took nearly an hour of crying shouting and screaming for Hayley to get onto a climbing wall and give it a go. I held my position knowing full well that she was going to get on that wall before the end of the session and she did. And the next time we went she went right on and up over the top. Whoop whoop go me!!

Yes, this is me celebrating the littlest wins for myself, this is something I could never do. I never saw anything I did as a win, but I now know if you want to bring change to your brain and be able to move forward into new things, you have to show your brain that you are winning, and this helps release the right chemicals to help you keep moving forward and not get stuck in the past. I want Hayley to know how to celebrate her wins, I have taught myself to say well done, you're doing a good job! And this is important because relying on other people to give us some sort of acknowledgement of our wins is dangerous and soul destroying when it doesn't happen.

This I believe is a hangover from the school system we go through in the UK, and even how we bring children up. A human's brain is negatively bias, so it will always see the bad and this is what we act on with our children.

It takes making a decision to see the good things that our children do and praise them on. It isn't easy, but it is doable to become present enough in a situation to notice these precious little things, which add up to bigger things in the future.

And it's the most rewarding thing I have learnt to do because nothing melts my heart more than Hayley saying thanks mum, I love you from the bottom of her heart not just because she thinks she should. Me positively praising Hayley results normally in a positive affirmation for me from Hayley, not always at the same time but again I choose to be receptive when she does love on me.

If I am honest my brain is still trying to tell me I am a crap mum sometimes, and that I am a failure at everything, it even did it today, but I get to choose to trust the process I am in. I get to choose what I think about myself, and I want Hayley to think good thoughts of herself so therefore as her biggest role model, I have to think and say good things about myself. I am a work in progress, and probably will still be when it's time for me to leave and go home to Heaven.

CHAPTER SEVENTEEN

The power in our words, I have already touched on the fact that I had an anger problem and I had taught and shown Hayley that anger was the answer to any difficult situation. I wanted to go a bit deeper with the subject because I know many parents can struggle with anger and it's a powerful emotion that when used in the wrong context goes from being a sign to us that all is not well, to a situation where others as well as yourself can be really hurt. The saying "sticks and stones may break my bones, but words will never hurt me" is the biggest load of nonsense. Mainly because it's a big fat lie. If you break a leg, it gets better hopefully, you think nothing more about it. It's a hindrance for a while trying to get around but that's about it.

Words said in anger on the other hand is a completely different kettle of fish because words can cut through us like a knife, especially if we harbour unhealed wounds already. In fact, we have an uncanny way us human beings of being able to know the weaknesses of another, and it is those weaknesses we use against them to cause the most damage. You see this happens in children, they see the weakness and they go for the jugular. It is because children tell the truth, the issue is the other child doesn't always have any rational thinking to be able to say, "I know I have that issue; I must get help to stop it being my reality" or have the words to be able to respond to the child and get them to stop.

I had it at school because I was overweight aged 10. I was 10 and 10 stone basically, and one delightful little boy decided to point that out to me one day, after they did that painful thing of writing everyone's height and weight on the board. This causing a barrage of negative self-talk that I spoke over myself every single day for over 20 years. It still tries to pop back into my thinking as a way of distracting me from doing anything that I want to do in life. My weight has been my nemesis for a very long time.

The brain works like this, "I think I want to write a book to help women", and my brain says "oh no don't do that you haven't lost enough weight yet". I think I want to go horse riding because I used to love it. "You can't go horse riding you're too heavy". I need some new clothes, "well you best stick to the usual because your thighs are still too fat really". I dread to think how the words of that lad and myself have stopped me doing hundreds of things in my life. I probably just upset him somehow, or he was having a bad day that's all, but I didn't have the rational thinking process at 10 to know any different. I have seen Hayley do exactly the same, something can be said and she will blow it out of context. It is only when I am there and can explain the situation that she is able to see what really happened.

I bet right now you can think of the exact words someone has spoken over you in the past that still come back to haunt you. You see words are powerful, and we throw them around without ever really thinking about it. Imagine if verbal abuse had the same punishment of going to prison as sexual assault or murder even. The truth is that's how damaging our words can be towards others or ourselves. We don't think to get help from the words which have been spoken over us from whoever has said them. If we have a physical injury, we go to the hospital or to a doctor. Mental and emotional injuries though, we just keep pushing deep inside ourselves making more and more soul clutter, until our bodies can't take it any longer. We either end up with long term disease or we struggle with mental health problems, depression, anxiety, psychosis, addictions including to food, which has been my biggest one.

When Hayley was 18 months old, she started to push all the right buttons to make me shout. I started to use anger, believing that was the best way to discipline a child. I would shout, I would get so angry sometimes I would throw things, I even threw her dolls pushchair one day and bent it. What a grown up I was being! This was because I was trying to control her through fear, manipulation, and anger.

She soon learnt though how to rebel and control me in return. The words of my mother-in-law ringing in my ears, "You need to sort her anger against you out before she is 7 or you're in trouble." Hayley was attacking me physically, hair pulling, biting, kicking, shouting. All because I had taught her that anger was the answer, and I didn't know how to process my emotions properly. Here we come back to our child models our behaviour, my outward physical behaviour of throwing things wasn't learnt from my parents shouting. No, the physical movements of my arms came again from that lad calling me fat because when I got to secondary school and it started again I learnt that being bigger, and being a farming girl I could pack a pretty good punch, and so that's where I learnt to defend myself.

There we were, me in my late 20s fighting with my child. Had I have known then the power of my words, I would have saved myself a lot of heart ache and time having to learn to forgive myself. However, I've learnt a lot about the power of saying sorry, and it has done me no harm to model that to Hayley. In fact, she now can say sorry to me or others truly from the heart, rather than it being something, she does because she has been told to say sorry after every little event or misdemeanour, she has been part of.

We must learn to humble ourselves and say sorry to our kids, because if I hadn't, I can hand on heart say I would not have the relationship I have with Hayley now. We would still be having daily screaming matches rather than occasional ones. We are always going to mess up because we aren't perfect, and that's a powerful lesson for our kids to learn as well. We can however after our anger has left us choose to say sorry, and explain what happened in us so then our children will learn how to regulate themselves before getting to that point.

The thing I am most glad about is that through my ability to learn new ways of thinking its created new ways for me to behave. I am setting Hayley up to be able to control her big emotions in a healthy way, not go in or out and cause more damage. As I watch her grow up this is what I am proud of myself for and what I hope you can see is possible, if you are struggling with your relationships with anyone, not just your children.

A personal experience.

The power in my words came into stark reality when Hayley was having a bad day, and she said the words "I wish I was dead". She was about 6, and I had been practising a lot of how to hold a safe space for these types of things to come out of her, without me getting emotional, I have become her personal Neuro-coach.

I repeated the words back to her and she had no idea why she had said them, or why she even thought it. I thought for a while, and I remembered that I was often in a dark place whilst pregnant and when she was little. I knew in that moment she was repeating the words I had said over myself whilst I was pregnant with her. I had wished myself dead probably multiple times because I was so miserable, I had never said it or thought it towards her, but it had become a belief in her as well. This was a shock to me and something I was truly sorry about, and it's this very thing that I can pray to God about purely because I didn't mean it to happen, but I don't always know what to do to make it better. Since then, Hayley has never said this again, and I really am grateful for that, because as a mother those words hurt.

And that my dear friend is how much our words affect our children, and how they would have affected us as children as well. Now we have a choice, we can discover the reasons why we are speaking such things in the first place, out of the mouth the heart speaks. This is where I have had a lot of coaching to uncover the hidden beliefs that I had harbouring in my mind.

I have also learnt to coach myself by writing out lots and lots of things that I say have come to the surface. These things I don't really want to share with other people, its private and I like to keep it that way. It is our belief systems that have been created over all of our lives, and even generationally that cause us to speak things we don't always want to speak, or take actions on things that give us either good or bad results. When I realised I could change any of my old belief patterns, and renew them with new ones I knew 100 percent I was onto a winner and it has been life changing.

CHAPTER EIGHTEEN

Neuroscience and brain-based coaching. I want to explain a little bit about Neuroscience and the amazing discoveries that people far cleverer than me have made when it comes to the human brain. It would seem that what has kept us humans alive for millennia is the ability to adapt to changing environments. We have the ability to see a problem and come up with a solution. God gave us the ability to keep ourselves safe by putting in a fight, flight freeze response system so should we ever get chased by a bear, we can get ourselves out of the situation hopefully.

Now we live in a different kind of world though, we have evolved, we can grow more food in one place and don't have to move around anymore. Most of the man-eating animals are only in certain areas of the world or no longer exist. Yet our brains and mine in particular have the ability to still go into fight or flight regularly if not all the time for no apparent reason. This we are seeing in sufferers of mental health blips such as anxiety, depression, psychosis, schizophrenia and more. I have experienced this myself, and have come to the realisation that I have been chronically stressed for years, and this is probably the cause of my weight gain and inability to get it off again. My brain has decided at some point that the world is always dangerous and I need to have cortisol and adrenaline running though me most, if not all of the time.

This has happened because the brain functions using our thoughts, or another word is neuropath-ways. These thoughts have been created through observations of the world around us, trial and error like learning to walk, they have come through what our family, teachers, friends have spoken to us, or even what has been spoken in the family and you think the child isn't aware of. These thoughts can come from all sorts of places. They are essentially voices in your head which has been perceived as a weird thing in the past, but the reality is many if not all people can have voices in their heads.

Neuroscience has helped us to understand that in order for us to function, and do what we want or need to do, we first have to have the thoughts to do it. Thoughts are how everything comes into being. This was how God first created the world, He thought about it and then he spoke everything into being. Now when we have a problem, we think about it and come up with a solution, to go ahead and solve the problem. Take a hoover for example, we didn't always have them but someone somewhere saw a problem, we needed to clean up a lot, and decided to make it easier. Now we have robot vacuum cleaners that do it for us.

Like I explained before I noticed I had all these voices in my head and that is what was making me so tired, what my head was saying weren't useful things that helped me solve problems. No, they were things that were stopping me solving problems, and ultimately stopped me doing what I desperately wanted to do and that was be a good mum, and help run a successful farming business so we can stay farming our farm for years to come, without worrying all the time about money.

My over stressed cortisol addicted run-away brain was out of control and since learning about neuroscience and becoming a Neuro-coach myself, I have realised there is massive potential in our own brains that we are just missing out on. It's like our brains have become so disorganised. I see my brain as a library and all of the books, thousands of them, were in a pile on the floor, and all the shelves were empty. There was no organisation, no way of recalling the useful information because it was a mess. What Neuro-coaching has done it has given me a way of organising the books, or rather my thoughts so that my brain has become more efficient. I no longer think I am busy all the time this is a big one, and I have made so much extra time in my days that people see me as being really busy, but I am not really, things are just organised differently so I am more productive. I have way more energy since literally working through each of my negative thought processes and deleting and rewiring them to be what I want them to be, to actually be useful.

The other interesting thing about the brain is, as I mentioned before is it's always trying to keep you safe and it can only do this by things you have experienced in the past. This is why if you want to try something different in life, you can struggle because your brain could literally throw up a thought like, "you're not good enough to do that" which then creates an emotional response learnt from the past and it stops you. This is where procrastination comes from. You can keep putting something off because your brain is perceiving it as something different or a challenge and it doesn't want you to do it.

It's weird when you think about it because I think we just think our brain is our brain and that's that. But actually, our brain is like plastic which is where the word neuroplasticity comes from and this means it can be changed, just like a computer can be coded and made to do what we want it to, so can our brains. It's just the world we are currently in is so driven by chaos it takes asking for help, or learning about it to be able to do anything. Which is why I get so excited about helping my clients through Neuro-coaching, because it is brain-based coaching that helps you discover what it is you want your life to look like, and then create the results using your own brain. I am just the person that helps you to see what you are thinking and notice what keeps you stuck.

When I realised that it was my own brain that was stopping me doing all the things my heart wanted me to do, it was stopping me feeling like I was a good mum, it was making me feel like I was a failure, like I wasn't good enough. I wasn't taking care of myself at all because my brain was telling me I wasn't good enough to spend the time on. My own brain has been wired against me for years, because of emotional traumas and wanting to protect myself which has been fine. It kept me safe, but it wasn't making me happy, I had no peace, I had no joy, my own brain was crushing me little by little and now I know there is a way to change that, and my whole life has changed. I am literally becoming a new person every day.

Sure I still make mistakes, because I need to, that bit won't stop as trial and error is something that humans need to progress in the world. But I am way more organised, I am not always rushing, I think and feel like a good mum and will say that to others, with not one ounce of guilt. I am a better wife than I was because I am more settled in myself for the greater part, and I can help Andrew in life by taking care of Hayley for us. And I can run the farm with a clearer mind, knowing and believing that I am supposed to be farming, with mum, dad and Andrew, but farming from a place of peace and health, rather than chaos and disease.

Another interesting fact about the brain is that it always wants to conserve energy, which is why it creates beliefs so rather than keep everything in our short-term memory, if we think a thought repetitively the brain decides to put it into the unconscious part of our brain, and it becomes a belief or a necessary thought that we need to survive. This is the same place that tells us to breathe, digest, blink, this part of the brain is running 90 percent of our day-to-day life. Can you imagine the energy you would need to remember to beat your heart, breathe, blink your eyes all day every day? So now think about what energy is being used by the brain when its full of negative not useful thoughts, and these are running your day. Now do you see why you can be so tired, yet you haven't necessarily done anything to be tired? Can you see how this can literally go on for years and essentially keep getting worse until you find a new piece of information, like in a book that makes you think this makes sense now?

We have super computers sitting on top of our shoulders, which we are only using a small piece of because that small piece has become so chaotic it thinks there isn't room for anything else in there.

Yet it is available to anyone who has the ability to read or listen and to learn about the brain to be able to rewire it. We have the knowledge now, we know how children's brains develop, we know what can happen if we don't hit certain developmental markers because we have had some kind of trauma happen in childhood.

We know that the brain can change, and thoughts are capable of being rewired. But the one thing that may stop you is the fear of change, the fear of changing things to make them better, especially when we are talking about the brain and the brain seems like something that shouldn't be tampered with.

Yet if you keep finding yourself coming up against a brick wall, especially when it comes to doing even the menial of tasks like tiding the house, the chances are your brain has gotten chaotic and that is creating a chaotic environment around you. This I found is what I was doing. I was actually creating an untidy house, which I then would get angry about because I would have to tidy it, but ultimately, I was making it untidy, and there was a way I could change my thoughts so that I could keep it more organised and spend less time cleaning, win win.

CHAPTER NINETEEN

I believe now more than ever that we are living in a broken world, I believe that we were originally created in love and peace but through choices we all make we live full of fear and chaos. Fear affects our energy levels and the energy of those around us. Fear steals, kills and destroys our relationships and essentially our lives. It is the fear that we all harbour inside of us, no matter how strong, that causes us to become controlling and angry unless you learn that the way you are currently doing things may not be all that good for you, or your family, you will never come into the reality that you have the power to change everything.

We right now have the power to change the reality for the next generation, right now you and I can vow to go on the journey to change things for our children and even for our family and friends. I have just given you a look into the reality that if you know and feel that the way you behave is not how you want to be, you have the power to make the choice and change. We can't change anyone else, we can't change our kids, our parents, our friends but we can change ourselves.

Personal story

Forgiving people who have hurt me in the past has been by far the hardest but most freeing experience I have ever had. I harboured a lot of bitterness towards people particularly my dad because of the time he spent on the farm, or rather because of the farm as an entity, it seemed when I was growing up it was all about the farm and not about me basically.

This bitterness came out in my words and actions toward him, and sadly it also come out onto people who were nothing to do with the farm. They were the worst mornings, waking up with a hangover thinking oh no, I punched that guy last night or not remember what I had said. There was one I couldn't even say sorry too because I had no idea who he was. I was just so angry all the time, it tied me up in knots it felt like, and I had no healthy way of letting go. These old belief systems and hurts can keep us trapped in the past and keeps projecting the past, into our future.

I have had to get help with my deep rooted unforgiveness, this for me is where my faith has really come into my life and changed things, because I can rewire my brain using neuro-coaching. But I needed healing on a deeper level, on a level that I couldn't change myself. I have had a lot of prayer and I have had counselling which has helped me to forgive people I thought I would never be able to, however I know now that the counselling opened things up too much for me at the time, and that doesn't need to happen to be able to move forward. I haven't had to do any big declarations to people or write anyone a letter. Using the information I have learnt from the bible about renewing the mind, and then what I have learned from science about our brain, thoughts and emotions I have been able to get the emotions and thoughts out of my soul one way or another, so they no longer have any power over me. Crying and sometimes sobbing has become my new best friend, because I know once I've processed it through tears, I will feel so much better. My old wounds have become scars, and I can talk about them now without getting upset, and this also means they are no longer running or ruining my life.

I remember listening once to a man who was an expert in brain trauma, and he had a client who was in a bombing. Over the course of 5 years the ladies life went to ruins because her brain was waiting for a bomb to go off. It was in a constant state of fight or flight, causing stress and severe mental health problems. This can be the case for anything that happens that has not been expected. Sudden death, sexual abuse, physical abuse, accidents. Our brains main job is to keep us safe; the problem is it is trying to keep us safe from something that may never happen again, and what fascinated me the most is we attract more incidents to ourselves to make more horrible situations happen.

What we believe and think is what we create. It is the biblical law of sowing and reaping, if we sow in fear, then we reap more fear. Overcoming the fear through rewiring our thoughts is how we change this narrative.

Our subconscious beliefs are attracting the negativity, I attracted and caused so much trauma to myself in the form of verbal abuse, that at 25 my physical body gave up completely and broke. The weight of my negative thoughts and emotions towards myself had that much of an impact on my body, our bodies keep the score. If we want to create lasting change, we have to be willing to create it from the inside out. The world is all about putting things into our bodies, changing our diets, doing exercise routines, taking supplements. But to get real change we have to be learning to catch what we are thinking and believing and change this.

A big part of what I teach Hayley now is, how she can choose what she allows in and what she doesn't. That unforgiveness does more damage to us than it does to the person we choose not to forgive. They are showing this to be true in the recovery of patients who have been in an accident, where another person caused it. If you don't know you need to forgive them for causing you the harm, then it can prolong your healing time. Your body wasn't intended to carry unforgiveness, bitterness guilt and shame. Which are all emotions that can have an effect on your overall health eventually.

If we have bitterness in our hearts, we can look like someone sucking a lemon, because our face shows what our hearts are feeling. You know exactly the face I mean, don't you? I reckon I wore that face a lot for a long time, scowling.

I have the kind of face which gives away my feelings without even saying a word. It works well if you are trying to frighten someone into submission, but it's not so great if you are wanting to allow someone to say what they need to say and there be no judgement from you. Hayley will often say to me, "stop judging me mum" even if I haven't said anything it's all in my facial expression.

CHAPTER TWENTY

I'm a farmers daughter at heart. It's a standing joke in our family that I was always running away through my teen years. I used to pack a bag, back then we had big brown leather bags. Dad would help me carry it into the car and by the time we got there we had chatted it out and I never really ran away. There were times I used to choose to stay at our family friends farm and work through the holidays, just because it seemed easier. I enjoyed the work, they had nearly 2000 sheep so there was lots of jobs to do, but I also enjoyed not having the pressure of being around my own farming family.

Looking back, I've always enjoyed farming, working on other people's farms, but when it came to my own it was a real drag, I wanted to live in town with my friends, walk to the shops and get a bus anywhere. That was how I saw living in a town, a place of freedom. How wrong I was because looking back now, especially through Covid, right where I am living in the middle of nowhere, but only 5 minutes from a main road really is the best place I can be.

It's only in the last few months that I have realised I really need to embrace my identity as a farmer's daughter and a woman in the farming industry, because I can see that I have been strategically placed for such a time as this. Where many are seeing the end of farming, I am seeing a whole new era, new opportunities, new technologies, healthier soil, plants, animals and humans. In fact, I would go as far as saying that I may not know what the future looks like, but I sure know that it will need to involve food, clean water and clean air. The three things that as a woman in farming I can help produce and contribute towards to ensure the people of Britain become healthier.

Lets face it, with an NHS on the brink of explosion, several million people relying on medications instead of revaluating their health through their lifestyle, we as farmers have a much bigger job to do.

We need to be learning to have a better lifestyle and health ourselves and then going out and showing others how to do that as well. There is a huge disconnect between people and their food, people and their health even, we aren't taking responsibility for our own health anymore. Instead, we are trusting that others namely doctors have all the answers to our problems, when they in fact don't. Our NHS is crumbling and is going more and more towards privatisation all the time.

I hear stories of people having to go home for 24 hours and be an outpatient to get their gallbladder removed, yet if they were private it would have been done on the day. I see women, my mum is one of them, who have been under intense stress for years trying to hold things together and do everything they can for their family and in the process, lose their own health and end up on 4 or 5 different medications for her thyroid, diabetes, cholesterol, blood pressure.

All conditions that are signs of burn out and too much stress that she didn't think she had. Fortunately for my mum we have a plan to get her off the medications again working from an inside out coaching approach, yet many will just keep taking the medication and need more medication to fight the symptoms. We should be able to listen to our bodies and know what we need to do to prevent getting sick. Instead, we are running ourselves into the ground before we wake up and realise, we need to do something about it. The stress of the way we live is slowly killing us, we are too over stimulated, it's like our brains are moving so fast they are starting to smoke, because they are full of thoughts we don't even need to be in there.

We rely so heavily on doctors, nurses, dentists, school teachers, always looking to other people to shift the blame onto if something goes wrong. It's not their fault it's our own for not listening to the natural rhythms of our body in the first place.

This isn't a new thing, this has been happening over the last 3-4 generations. We have disconnected from ourselves, and every generation and it gets worse because children model their adults. Add in the technological age we are currently living in which has its good and bad sides, and we have a walking disaster zone. It was having Hayley and learning from her that I have been able to see that I want this toxic cycle of always looking to other people for the answers to stop.

I wanted to know my own body and what was going on in it, to help myself to become healthier and know what steps it is I need to take. And most of all I wanted to teach Hayley how to tune in to her own body. To ask herself why I am feeling like this? and for her to know and do something about it. To be able to choose a healthier path forward with her connecting into her mind, body and soul, so she doesn't end up like me, aged 25 and so broken she can't function.

In the Western World it seems we find it impossible to tap into our intuition to know just what it is our body needs from food, to sleep and everything else. That's because we live in a country that needs an economy to function, and that economy is running on medication, non-foods, broken relationships and a whole heap of unhealthy spending habits. I believe farming and good quality food and water should be the backbone of the economy and this is where things are going horribly wrong.

It's not about people being healthy and living great lives. The focus is about people making money and living unhealthy lives because of it. You take money out of the equation, and you get left with people who still need to survive, and need to be healthy to keep providing for their family. They need to know how to be able to do that without relying on what's always been there. Like supermarket shelves full of food, and especially highly processed foods which are empty calories with no real nutritional values.

I stopped looking at the outside world for answers to how I needed to improve my health and started looking inside instead, and the results have been rather incredible. As a 5th generation farmers daughter, I believe I have the privilege of being passed down many skills that I need for farming, and even for health and restoring the farm from the years of taking from it and not replacing. We may just have to go backwards to be able to go forwards, especially when it comes to soil and being able to restore it. Then the plants, animals and humans become healthier. For me its started by asking myself questions about my own health, and then how we can make the farm a healthier and happier place.

I stand in our fields a lot and I stop to observe things more. The issue was I had a whole heap of beliefs and stories that I have believed that have been passed down, which aren't true, or they are just not relevant for now and have actually been mistakes that have been made that we get to choose to learn from, and change.

This is what I think has happened since World War 1 and 2, the government took over to stop the nation starving and we never really stopped looking to them for the answers, and the next steps of what to do. And look where that has got us! So now here I am on a journey of clearing out my belief system to be able to farm in a way that not only serves my family but other families around us as well, to all become healthier and happier, to be thriving not just surviving.

You see farms aren't supposed to be places devoid of people, in fact they are supposed to be places of community, places to come and receive healing mentally, emotionally, or physically and places where there is such a sense of family you just feel like you belong even if you aren't destined for farming. Instead, farms have become places of fear and worry of "what could happen". They have become places for lone wolfing meaning on many farms it's just one person doing everything, because everyone must go out to work, even the one person deemed as the main farmer sometimes, because the finances just are not there to support families, this is really sad.

I have always been one to have parties, to get people onto the farm, to have people for coffee, or lunch or a sit by the river. Rare chances for people who don't have farms to come and experience them. I always believed I did these things to get out of the "actual" farming, but I do these things to share this beautiful piece of Devon, I am able to call my home with others. It's meant to be shared! Opening it up even further now to families to come on farm tours has been even more important because we are able to teach people about farming, and ultimately give them snippets of how they can be healthier, by reconnecting them to the land and their food source.

These are the things that light me up, these are the things I love to do, but because farming seems to have become a crazy health and safety zone, we stopped opening up, for fear something bad will happen. Which is no longer happening on our farm, as we open up to families and to adult groups to give farm tours, covering everything from soil to cow poo, to beef production and everything in between. The tours we have done have been brilliant and given us all back a buzz, even my dad, who at times can be the most worried about it all.

We as farmers should be amongst some of the healthiest people in the world, we spend our lives in green spaces, in fresh air, moving, eating good food we have produced. Yet when I look around me all I see is physical pain, new knees and hips, anger, and a bunch of old men who really have done their time and they either need to learn to let go or find someone who is going to be willing to farm in a new way. To make sure this little island of the UK with far too many people on it can feed and water everyone.

CHAPTER TWENTY ONE

I have no real idea how I have still ended up back here, other than if it's a divine calling then it's a divine calling. I didn't want to be here farming until now, but here I am. I know it's part of what I am supposed to be doing, I married well because my husband was born to farm with no family farm. Which means now I get to do what I really want to do and that's to help you. Help you reach your full potential, be the present mum, to have more time in your day, to bring healing to your relationships, to design a business that is going to give you back more than what you put in just like farms should.

Right now you are reading this for a reason, and whether the next step is to work with me or to find someone else to help you move forward, you need to do it. Your 1% in the world has never been more important and the longer you leave it undiscovered, the longer those who are waiting for YOU to discover YOU must wait.

Come join me on the path to a better life, If you want to find out how you can take the next steps with me get in touch today **thedevonshireshepherdess@outlook.com**

Printed in Great Britain
by Amazon